Weight Loss

Successful 10-Day Ayurvedic Detox Diet And Weight Loss Program

By Michael Dinuri

COPYRIGHT © 2015 BY MICHAEL DINURI. ALL RIGHTS RESERVED

This document is geared towards providing exact and reliable information in regards to the topic and issue covered. The publication is sold with the idea that the publisher is not required to render accounting, officially permitted, or otherwise, qualified services. If advice is necessary, legal or professional, a practiced individual in the profession should be ordered.

- From a Declaration of Principles which was accepted and approved equally by a Committee of the American Bar Association and a Committee of Publishers and Associations.

In no way is it legal to reproduce, duplicate, or transmit any part of this document in either electronic means or in printed format. Recording of this publication is strictly prohibited and any storage of this document is not allowed unless with written permission from the publisher. All rights reserved.

The information provided herein is stated to be truthful and consistent, in that any liability, in terms of inattention or otherwise, by any usage or abuse of any policies, processes, or directions contained within is the solitary and utter responsibility of the recipient reader. Under no circumstances will any legal responsibility or blame be held against the publisher for any reparation, damages, or monetary loss due to the information herein, either directly or indirectly.

Although the author and publisher have made every effort to ensure that the information in this book was correct at press time, the author and publisher do not assume and hereby disclaim any liability to any party for any loss, damage, or disruption caused by errors or omissions, whether such errors or omissions result from negligence, accident, or any other cause. This book is not intended as a substitute for the medical advice of physicians. The reader should regularly consult a physician in matters relating to his/her health and particularly with respect to any symptoms that may require diagnosis or medical attention.

Respective authors own all copyrights not held by the publisher.

The information herein is offered for informational purposes solely, and is universal as so. The presentation of the information is without contract or any type of guarantee assurance.

The trademarks that are used are without any consent, and the publication of the trademark is without permission or backing by the trademark owner. All trademarks and brands within this book are for clarifying purposes only and are the owned by the owners themselves, not affiliated with this document.

Table of Contents

Why I Wrote This Book 1

Why You Should Read This Book 5

Chapter 1: Ayurveda—A Path To Perfect Health 9

Chapter 2: The Ayurvedic Way To Fight Fat 21

Chapter 3: Ayurvedic Detox Programs 33

Chapter 4: Day By Day Easy Program to Follow 45

Chapter 5: How To Lose Weight With Ayurveda And Maintain It 57

Conclusion 71

About the Author 75

Why I Wrote This Book

Ayurveda is an important branch of treatment for various kinds of ailments that are related to your body and health. Of course everyone wants to remain fit and healthy. There are some people who are very conscious about their diet and weight. These are the people who pay attention to the food that they eat but are still not aware of the reasons behind the increase in their weight. Ayurveda has so much importance in our daily lives, but most people are not fully aware of the benefits which it will provide them. I have written this book to increase the knowledge of Ayurveda so that people may be able to act upon the golden tips of Ayurveda and thus attempt to get rid of so many problems which plague their health.

Due to a lack of knowledge about Ayurveda, people often fail to act upon the way they should in order to treat their health problems. So I have written this book as a package of ayurvedic information which will work as a guide for all those who are looking for the related information and who want to get adequate ayurvedic knowledge so that they can get the ultimate benefits out of it no matter whatever their circumstances may be.

Your lifestyle and the way by which you behave with the people around you also plays an important role in determining the extent to which you remain healthy and fit. Think of it as karma—if you remain nice to others you will get courtesy in return as well. So I have written this book to tell you the importance of your everyday lifestyle in determining your health.

When you do Ayurveda to get a better life, you must think of a diet which will help you get rid of extra fat and also detoxify your body of all the toxic substances which has accumulated inside your body. If these don't get eliminated, these toxins will prove to be very harmful to you. So I have added proven steps in this book to make you aware of various ways toxins can accumulate inside your body. One of the purposes of writing this book is to make you aware of the various ways using Ayurveda can get rid of toxins and help you lead a healthy life without any problems.

The basic purpose of writing this book is to make you fully aware of Ayurveda and all its related terms which you should know when you are looking for various ways which can help you not only in understanding Ayurveda but also to implement it properly.

Why You Should Read This Book

This book is a package for all those who are looking to learn about Ayurveda and all information related to it. This is a practical guide to all those who are seeking information regarding Ayurveda and are interested in being healthy and fit by following the tips as given by the ayurvedic way of treating them. These days more and more people are looking for information about how Ayurveda can help treat their particular ailment.

There is a lot of information which is available publically for everyone about the latest ayurvedic treatments and methods, but there is a real scarcity of sincere advice on how to use these ayurvedic medicines in one's daily life and the possible benefits which can be taken out of it. So if you are looking for some sincere advice on working with ayurvedic medicines and the ways it can treat ailments, then you should read this book completely so that you won't miss any information regarding Ayurveda and how you can lose your weight with the help of an ayurvedic approach.

One of the very important aspects which are associated with Ayurveda is that it has the ability of understanding and defining various kinds of subtle energies which reside within your body. If you want to learn everything about those energies, then you should completely go through this book because it will help you get all the related information you desire.

By using Ayurveda for prevention, you can save yourself from becoming the victim of so many health-related problems. Many chronic diseases can also be avoided by using this type of treatment and this book is one of the best sources from which you can get the best information regarding the ways you can avoid them. Detox may help you out in preventing many diseases and losing your weight so that you will have a healthier lifestyle when you opt for detoxification through Ayurveda.

This book is basically a treasure of ayurvedic knowledge which should be a part of everyone's life so that whenever anyone needs a solution to any problem related to health, they can get information regarding that using this book. In addition to improving the health of the mind and soul, ayurvedic medicines also help in losing excess body fat. So if you are looking to lose your weight, you would be happy to know that you can easily do so by using the ayurvedic medicines. This book contains all the proven steps and strategies which you should use to get the right condition of your health without any problems or hurdles.

A continuous process of repairing and renewal takes place inside your body and understanding that process is very important for everyone. As the process of repairing and renewal goes on, metabolic wastes are produced naturally inside our body and the process of eliminating these wastes must be carried out effectively so that you may feel healthy and no health-related problem can harm you. So to avoid these kinds of problems all you should do is look for the related information in this book and forget all the worries which you have in your life.

I hope that I have added enough reasons why you should grab this book and the benefits this book can be to you as it is a set of information related to Ayurveda. If you are looking to learn the basics and tips to incorporate Ayurveda in your daily life, then all you have to do is look keenly at all the steps which have been added in this book in order to avoid any sort of problem or ailment related to your health.

Chapter 1: Ayurveda—A Path To Perfect Health

What is Ayurvedic Medicine?
Several thousand years ago, the sages of India developed Ayurveda, which is one of the most powerful and first forms of medicine in the world. Ayurveda has been used in India to promote the health and balance of the body's basic energies and rhythms of nature. The origin of Ayurveda is Indian, but the use of the healing practice is used worldwide because of its effective healing practices. Ayurveda is more than a simple system of treating illness; it is a science of life. The word itself means "Ayur" equaling "life" and "veda" equaling "knowledge." "Veda" can also mean "science."

The primary focus of Ayurvedic medicine is to promote good health, rather than fight disease. Ayurveda provides us with the knowledge of how to prevent disease and how to eliminate its root cause if it occurs. The emphasis is on the entirety—where the body is not separated from the soul. It is based on the belief that health and wellness depend on a subtle balance between the mind, body, and spirit. This technique helps the individual bring out the body's own self-healing ability and to eliminate the reasons for illness and unbalance in the body. Healthy people can also benefit from Ayurveda since it can also be used as a preventative technique. Ayurveda places great importance on lifestyle, eating habits, and daily routines. Ayurveda also guides one on how to fine-tune their lifestyle based on the change of seasons.

In addition to improving the health of the mind and soul, ayurvedic medicines also help you lose body fat. So if you are looking to lose your weight, you would be happy to know that you can easily use ayurvedic medicines to obtain your goal.

Theory of Ayurveda

Use of ayurvedic medicines is actually based on a theory about the universe and its elements. It says that everything in this universe is connected to another thing by one way or another. It is not mandatory that the thing be living or non-living. Each and every thing in the entire universe is related to one another. The same should also be true of your mind, soul, and body.

The theory clearly says that when your mind, body, and soul are connected to each other and with the universe as well, it will lead to good health—not only physically, but mentally and spiritually as well. There should be no disruption in all of these elements of anyone's life because any kind of break in the connection would lead to poor health conditions.

Not having a lot of fat in your body is also a sign of good health, and if you are obese you will definitely be considered as one who has bad health. So if you want to get rid of the extra body fat you have, there should be a good harmony between your mind, body, and soul so that you may enjoy good health along with the benefits of losing extra fat.

What Things Can Cause Disruptions?
The theory of Ayurveda says that any disruption in the connection between the mind, body, and soul can lead to unhealthy conditions, but the point to ponder is: what are those things which can cause disruptions? Anything of any kind which directly or indirectly affects your comfort level can lead to your imbalance with your connection to the universe. According to this theory, the following are the things which can cause disruptions in your well-being:

- Any kind of injuries
- Defects which are genetic
- Age factor
- Changes in climate or seasons
- Abrupt changes in emotions

The Workings of Your Body
The constitution of your body in terms of Ayurveda is called "prakriti." The working of your body so that you remain heathy and fit depends upon the unique combination of some characteristics which are not only physical but also psychological. This entire working of your body and its constitution which comes from the combination of physical and psychological attributes is the prakriti. There is a belief that it does not change throughout your life.

Basic Elements

As said by the ayurvedic theory, every person in this world is made of a combination of the five elements which are found in the universe, and these elements have a great impact on anyone's life. These five elements include:

1. Space
2. Air
3. Fire
4. Water
5. Earth

When all of these five elements are combined inside the human body, they in turn cause the formation of three basic forces which are sometimes considered as energies and are called "doshas." The main purpose of this life energy or "dosha" is to control the workings of your body perfectly and allow you to practice harmony among the various elements of your body. Thus, it can be said that these doshas are meant to control the connection between different life elements and help in avoiding the loss of harmony among them.

They include:

- Vata dosha (They are meant for space and air)

- Pitta dosha (They are meant for fire mainly)

- Kapha dosha (They are meant for water and earth)

Every person in this world is comprised of a combination of any of these doshas which are unique for each person. Among these three, usually one dosha appears to be dominant over the others. There should be a proper balance among all the doshas which a person is comprised of, according to Ayurveda theory. There is a belief that if these doshas get imbalanced, you get sick or your health lowers. This is because they are closely related to the proper workings of your body. The imbalance can be considered to be of long-term significance if no proper care is taken, which may lead it to transform into a severe chronical condition.

The Five-Element System of Ayurveda
I have already mentioned that there are five basic elements of the ayurvedic system: space, water, earth, air, and fire. Now go a bit more into detail on them.

Space/Ether (Akasha)
This element is considered to be the most delicate element among the five. Space is the area in which all universal objects exist. It has been discovered that space governs the part of the body which has empty places inside the atoms that our bodies are comprised of. The actions done by the mouth and our sense of hearing are also ruled by space. It has the qualities of subtle, clear, light, and soft.

Air (Vayu)
The rule which air follows is "movement." It is related to motion. It basically depicts the extent to which anyone's intent is affixed by looking for ways by which one can achieve their goals. Sense of touch in humans, the actions of hands, and the energy of the nervous system is governed by this element. It has the attributes of subtle, uneven, dry, and cold.

Fire (Agni)
The basic rule which fire follows is "metabolism." The balance of the temperature of the human body, aptitude, and knowledge is absolutely governed by this element. The process of food assimilation is also governed by fire in the human body as well as vision. Its association is commonly

known to be with the energy emitted from the sun. It has the attributes of sharp, hot, light, and subtle.

Water (Jala)
As water is the universal solvent, the main principle which water follows is "transportation." It is also present inside our body and carries the toxins away from the body's cells. We can say that it is the river of everyone's life. Sense of taste in humans is connected with this element. Now the association of water with the ayurvedic system is that it is believed that it has a great and firm association with the chemical energy produced inside our body. It has the attributes of oily, liquid, soft, cool, and dull.

Earth (Prithvi)
The earth is dominant at every place where there is stability and firmness. The main principle which is followed by earth is "structure." The function of earth is to support the creatures living on this world and to give them support. It is related to all the solid structures of the body such as teeth, skin, nails, cartilage, etc. The sense of smell and the process of excretion in humans are governed by this element. It has the attributes of dull, gross, hard, and hefty.

All of these elements can impart balance in your life when working together properly. If any of these elements gets out of balance, it would lead you towards discomfort, and as result, there can be a threat to your life as well. Each of these elements has properties which are related to various parts and functions of the body.

So it can be said that the ayurvedic system is entirely related to man and its universe and it can be considered as a science of self-healing as it involves you and the five universal elements to be in connection with one another. This must be achieved in order to make your health balanced and good and you'll also be able to lose your weight using the ayurvedic medicines, which will be discussed in a later chapter.

Overall, it can be said that the five basic elements of Ayurveda work completely for your benefit. Various combinations of these elements turn out to be three doshas which include the vata, pitta, and kapha, and they play supporting roles behind the workings of several functions of the body.

Vata
Vata is meant to support the motion or movement of the body as it is formed by the combination of space and air. It provides the body with the energy

needed for the proper functioning of the respiratory system, heartbeat, and the process of muscle contraction. The energy required for proper circulation of the blood in the body is also provided by vata.

Pitta

Pitta is comprised of fire only. The regulation of the body to have an effective control on metabolism is done by this vital presence of fire. The release of several kinds of hormones, heat production in the body, and the regulation of digestion is also carried out with the help of pitta. It is also responsible for converting the brain's impulses to proper thought patterns.

Kapha

Kapha is formed by the combination of water and earth and it is used basically as a lubricant throughout the body. Basic structures which include the muscles, skeleton, ligaments, organs, and many others are basically under the building block of kapha. It is also responsible for ensuring that the joints are working smoothly.

It can be said that the five elements of Ayurveda is a complete system by which the importance of ayurvedic medicines can be extracted and all of these elements in combination with one another help in gaining many benefits—even more than anyone's imagination.

Chapter 2: The Ayurvedic Way To Fight Fat

As a result of poor performance of the digestive system, various toxins are produced inside the human body. These toxins are called "ama," which are produced by the body. If the production of ama continues to build up within the body, it may lead to the creation of another more harmful poison called "amavisha," which may cause many diseases, including obesity.

How Are Toxins Produced?
Ama is just like a sticky substance which is usually produced as a result of the process in which food does not become fully digested. If you eat the wrong food or weaker digestion takes place, then it

would result in the production of a toxic substance called ama. The main cause of outbreak of ama is the low level of agni which may lead to low digestion and it happens when imbalances in agni take place.

Taking care of this toxin in your body is very important because if no proper care is taken, then it could lead to the formation of an even more severe type of toxin called amavisha, which can also cause the production of excess fat within the body, which may lead to obesity.

As the production of fat takes place due to ama, it may lead to the production of clogs in various channels inside the human body which are visible and can also cause the production of clogs in organs such as bronchi, lungs, arteries, liver, etc., which is not good for the overall health of anyone.

The most dangerous clog is in the arteries because when the fat produced due to ama gets deposited in the arteries, it may lead to blockage in one's blood circulation and as a result, the possibility of a heart attack may increase.

It is the belief of so many people who are overweight that although they are taking a kapha diet, they are not getting the desired results of their weight loss. In a kapha diet, it is recommended that whatever you eat should be made by using "dry cooking." That means if you are following the kapha diet, you can make your food by grilling, roasting, and baking, as all these methods are included in dry cooking. In addition to this, in a kapha diet, you use coconut oil instead of any other oil as it really helps in losing weight. Warm and spicy food can also be opted sometimes in a kapha diet if you want.

Use of dry foods help in increasing the amount of vata in the body which makes the amount of kapha balanced in the body. Foods that are light, dry, or warm are taken by a person who is opting for a kapha diet. Such a person should greatly avoid things like cold food and beverages.

One of the main causes of having ama is the increase in quantity of vata in the body, which may be due to the intake of an incorrect diet or due to having an incorrect lifestyle. As vata is air, it can be blown on fire and as a result of this, the fire gets imbalanced and ultimately the digestion process is affected which leads to the production of ama.

But what if a kapha diet fails to achieve the desired results? In the ayurvedic form of fighting against accumulated fats in the body as a result of several poisonous substances like ama, it is better to go to an ayurvedic physician.

Importance of Agni in Metabolism

Agni is responsible for the proper workings of the metabolic system of the body and if it fails, then it could lead to the formation of toxins like ama, which is the root cause of accumulation of excess fat inside the body. As already mentioned, ama is produced due to the improper digestion of food items, and as a result, weight increases. But if a person wants to get rid of excess fat using the ayurvedic way, then he should focus on it, which would help in getting rid of the excess body fat.

If you want to have healthy agni, then you must ingest food which is cooked fresh, can be digested easily, and has pure ingredients. Not only this, but you should take the meal at a proper time as taking a meal not at a proper time could also lead to malfunction of agni, which may lead to accumulation of fat in the body. You should eat when you're hungry and not wait, otherwise agni gets imbalanced. Also try not to eat heavy in the evening and close to your bed time. Always take care of your agni, which is very important.

In addition to the tips mentioned above, you should also try to act upon more ayurvedic tips to help yourself fight successfully against the problem of fat which has been accumulating inside your body.

Drink Warm Lemon Water
Drinking half a lemon or 2–3 tablespoons of fresh lemon juice in warm water can prove to be very beneficial for the proper functioning of your digestive system as this combination of warm water and lemon juice is enriched with vitamin C, which helps in making the body's pH balanced. This will also help in improving the process of digestion, which will prevent the production of ama inside the body. Thus, the first thing to do in the morning is to drink warm lemon water, then wait for at least 10–15 minutes before eating or drinking anything else.

Add Ayurvedic Tastes
In order to fight against excess fat of the body using Ayurveda, you must add six basic tastes of food at every meal which includes: sour, sweet, salty, pungent, bitter, and astringent tastes. These will help in balancing the appetite and the process of digestion in your body. Here are some of the examples of the six types of tastes which will help you decide what to eat.

SWEET
This includes whole grains, starchy vegetables, dairy, chicken, fish, sugar, honey, and molasses.

SOUR
Citrus fruits, berries, plums, tomatoes, pickled foods, vinegar, cheese, and yogurt.

SALTY
Any food to which table salt has been added.

PUNGENT
Peppers, onions, garlic, cayenne, black pepper, cloves, ginger, mustard, salsa, and chilies.

BITTER
Spinach, kale, sprouts, beets, bitter greens, turmeric, romaine lettuce, leafy greens, celery, and broccoli.

ASTRINGENT
Lentils, grape skins, cauliflower, figs, pomegranates, dried beans, green apples, and tea.

Make Your Dosha Balanced
To get your dosha balanced for your weight loss, you have to eat a balanced diet in several types of dosha. For example, to get the balance in the vata

type, you must eat something which is warm and heavy, for pitta you must eat something which is dry and cool, and for kapha you must eat something which is warm and light. By taking these food items in every dosha, you will be able to make it balanced and thus it will help in getting rid of excess fat.

This is how you can balance your dosha with a combination of various kinds of taste:

	Most Balancing	Most Aggravating
Vata	Sweet, Sour, Salty	Bitter, Pungent, Astringent
Pitta	Sweet, Bitter, Astringent	Sour, Salty, Pungent
Kapha	Pungent, Bitter, Astringent	Sweet, Sour, Salty

Maintain a Yoga Practice

To fight against excess body fat with the ayurvedic way, you must maintain a daily yoga practice. It will really help in winning the fight against obesity and excess weight.

While you incorporate all of the ayurvedic tips which I have mentioned above, by doing regular yoga exercise and by following the rule of keeping yourself happy, you can help yourself become healthy overall. The only thing which you need is to keep your metabolism balanced so that it will not lead to the production of ama, and ultimately, you will be far away from picking up weight.

It is highly recommend to do a yoga sun solution every morning just after you wake up. This can be learnt by taking classes for yoga. Proper instructions can only be received from a professional yoga instructor.

Bhastrika Pranayama for Weight Loss
You can opt for some breathing techniques in yoga called "pranayama," which will help you in getting the desired results of losing your excess weight. One of the most important and effective breathing exercises for losing your weight is the Bhastrika pranayama for weight loss.

It is considered to be the ultimate and most effective pranayama related to losing weight. It is related to power and energy. It will help you improve your metabolism at a cellular level so that it can promote health by burning the excess fat which you have accumulated.

This pranayama is also called "bellows breath," owing to the fact that it depicts the true working associated with bellows, which are used for fueling the fire. Its function is to pump the air and "life force" to the whole body.

- You can get an unlimited number of benefits by opting for Bhastrika pranayama for weight loss including the boosting of your metabolic rate so that it can promote the burning of your excess body fat faster.

- It helps in making your body purified by helping in the elimination of various toxins and harmful wastes.

- It assists in the generation of heat inside your body which will ultimately help in opening the pathways of energy needed by the body.

Not only this, but Bhastrika pranayama for weight loss enhances the fortification of your nervous system very effectively.

How Do You Do It?

- To do Bhastrika pranayama for weight loss, you must be in a comfortable position. You can do it by sitting, standing, or even by lying down, but a sitting posture is considered to be the best.

- First, you have to elongate the spine in an upward direction while at the same time you are lengthening your neck.

- Make an attempt to bring your chin back just like you are becoming attentive.

- Now close your eyes and place both of your hands on your knees, placing your palms up. While doing so, you should also relax the muscles of your stomach.

- Now it's time to breathe while applying the full force through your nostrils. While doing this, your emphasis on inhalation and exhalation should be equal.

- You should breathe in a way that when you exhale or inhale, the expansion and contraction of the diaphragm should be in conjunction with it.

- All of your breaths should be powerful and deep so that you may feel them. A steady rhythm is created by you while doing this.

- Both for inhalation and exhalation, the pace should be of about 1 second.

- Make an attempt to repeat the process 10 times. Then make an attempt to completely inhale followed by holding your breath for about 1–5 seconds.

- After doing this you have to completely exhale the breath and after doing so, you have completed one round.

- After that, a short break should be opted in order to make yourself relaxed and then continue with your work out for at least 5 rounds.

- By following the above mentioned steps, you will be making an attempt to bring a huge amount of energy in you, which will help you get rid of excess body fat by utilizing the principles of Bhastrika pranayama.

Ayurvedic Way of Getting Rid of Excess Body Fat

If a kapha diet fails in ridding excess body fat, then the only other ayurvedic way of getting rid of excess body fat is by burning all the fat using the powers of agni. Being overweight is not usually caused when kapha is in balance. The only way by which kapha gets imbalanced is when a person eats more than he requires or eats too much junk or too much fatty foods.

The main and important cause of gaining excess weight is ama, which will lead to an accumulation of excess fat in the body.

Chapter 3: Ayurvedic Detox Programs

If you have a poor lifestyle and make bad food choices, then it might be possible that as a result of this negligence, vital systems of your body will become imbalanced energetically. Not only this, but the enzymes that work to regulate the metabolism of your body get slowed down, and thus your capacity of digesting food will also be greatly affected. As a result of all these interrelated processes, whatever food you eat is not able to provide the essential nutrients, which are necessary for your body. Thus, your immune system also gets slowed down and may lead to the malfunctioning of various systems, especially the endocrine system inside your body.

Accumulation of Toxins Inside the Body

It is a fact that the state of repairing and renewal is constantly associated with the various functions of the body. While the process of repairing and renewal is going on, metabolic wastes are produced naturally inside our body and the process of elimination of these wastes must be carried out effectively so that you may feel healthy and no health-related problem can harm you. On a daily basis, our exposure to several types of pathogens such as viruses and bacteria also takes place and our immune system fights against these harmful pathogens to save our body from the adverse effects of all of these pathogens.

But if the digestive and immune system gets disturbed or weaker, it would allow the pathogens to attack your body and may leave many adverse and harmful effects.

Our bodies have the capacity to cope with various kinds of toxins up to a certain level but after reaching a certain level, the ability of our bodies to cope against adverse effects slows down and ultimately, the body fails to save itself from the harmful effects of all the toxins which are produced inside the body.

If you continuously opt to eat processed food, breathe polluted air, and continue to drink water which is not clean, then the level of toxins will reach up to the extent which your body cannot cope with easily. This situation can really prove to be an alarming situation for you and you should take some measures to detoxify your body so that these harmful toxins may not harm you anymore.

Building up of Ama (Toxins)

The toxins which are produced inside the body are called "ama." As soon as the toxins are built inside the body, they at once get transformed into a solid and crystalline form and these crystals then interfere with the normal functioning of the body tissues and act as a hurdle in the proper functioning of the body. Their ultimate effects include the hardening of not only the joints but of bones and muscles as well. Not only this, but it may also cause blockage in the arteries, and the digestive system also gets affected. If the digestion process is strong, then the toxins will not be able to harm the body due to the strong impact of the digestive system. The toxins will not be able to have any negative impact on the normal functioning of the body in any case.

It can be said that ama is basically the undigested food which later acts as toxic substances that are not good for our body. But Ayurveda will definitely help you get rid of these toxins from your body so that your body may not face any sort of harmful conditions. Ayurvedic detox is an effective way by which you can detoxify your body and live a really healthy life.

Panchakarma—The Purification of the Body

Panchakarma is normally done at an ayurvedic clinic. You can also do a small 10-day detox program at home, which is included in this book. If you are looking for a local ayurvedic clinic then you can consult a local directory or you can travel to India to do so. It is important that the process be done at a proper ayurvedic clinic. This is especially good for treating illness and reducing body fat. There is lot to be written about panchakarma; this information is very short. If you do not know what panchakarma is, then you must be aware of the fact that it is a word used for detoxification or purification of the body from harmful substances in the Sanskrit language. It is comprised of some actions which are necessary to be carried out when you are required to get rid of harmful substances from your body. These steps are considered crucial when you are about to make your body clean and purified from the toxins which are produced inside the body.

It is basically an ancient branch of Ayurveda which has been known for thousands of years due to its ability of making your body detoxified and help in improving not only your immune system, but other functions as well. It not only helps you in making your mind and body revitalized, but also assists in granting strength and balance to all the functions which are going on inside the body by taking the help from a wide variety of measures which are therapeutic in nature.

According to modern trends which are dominating in the process of panchakarma, using herbal concoctions will help a lot in detoxifying the body and thus help in making it fit and free of any kind of problem. All the toxins are eliminated out of the body and these toxins are not only water based but oil based as well. Both of these toxins are successfully eliminated from the body only with the help of panchakarma. From all the body parts which have an accumulation of toxins, the process of panchakarma can readily eliminate all kinds of toxins and thus no bodily issue remains behind. Once you get your tissues cleaned of all kinds of impurities, the food which you eat will effectively get metabolized and will really help in bringing improvements in your bodily health.

Benefits of Panchakarma

This process of making your body free of toxins is very helpful for living a healthy life, and by opting for this process you will get the following benefits:

- It helps in making your digestive tract clean and purified.

- It assists you in bringing energy and vitality in your body.

- It is a major source of making your mind balanced.

- It greatly helps in strengthening the immune system.

- With the help of panchakarma, you are able to reduce your stress and anxiety.

- The process of assimilation during digestion also gets improved.

- The free radicals inside your body which cause diseases are also eliminated.

- It helps in assigning strength to your endocrine system.

- Clarity of mind can be achieved by using this process.

- It helps in releasing all of your negative emotions.

- It helps in increasing the tone and strength of muscles up to a greater extent.

- It regulates and balances your nervous system.

- Panchakarma can work effectively and can reduce the amount of cholesterol in the blood.

- The bone tissues get strengthened and regenerate.

- It helps clear arteries.

- Low and high blood pressure become balanced.

- It helps in detoxifying the liver and blood.

- It increases the amount of happiness in your life.

- All the toxic metabolic wastes are easily excreted and eliminated from the body.
- It can also help in curing many diseases.

Foods to be Avoided During Panchakarma Treatment

When you are going through the detox program of panchakarma, you are required to totally eliminate the following foods from your daily routine. This is because these foods can jeopardize your heath and may impact negatively on the digestive and immune system of your body when it is going through the process of detoxification. All of these foods are known as "hard to be digested" when your digestive system is busy in an attempt to excrete all kinds of toxins out of your body. So it is strongly recommended that you not take the following foods during the process of panchakarma in any case. These things should be avoided:

- Canned and bottled soft drinks
- Confectionery items
- Frozen food
- Microwaved food
- Sour fruit salads
- Pasteurized milk

- Alcohol
- Coffee
- Caffeine
- Tamarind
- Cream
- Pasta bread
- Brown rice
- Vinegar
- Soy sauce
- Fish and red meats
- Canned food
- Melons
- Mushrooms
- Olives
- Onion
- Cold beverages and food

Thus, when you are going through the treatment of panchakarma, you are not allowed to have any of the foods mentioned above.

There are several types of therapies which are associated with panchakarma. The process of panchakarma is comprised of several steps and many kinds of treatments are being given to the person who is going through this process. One of the treatments is to have a massage of some light oil or any of the herbal oils which are available on the market. The time duration of these massage therapies varies from one type to another as there are so many therapies which are offered during the treatment of panchakarma; these therapies are tailor-made for each and every individual by an ayurvedic doctor. The purpose of the massage is to help the body lose the toxins which are produced inside the body and which are very harmful for the body if not excreted out.

Followed by the massage therapy, another therapy which can be taken into consideration is the "svedana" which involves the herbal stem therapy in order to make the channels of the body dilated and to help the impurities get mobilized so that they can be taken out of the body quickly and without any hurdles.

Another therapy which is done in addition to the massage therapy is "shirodhara," which helps make the mind relaxed and free of tension and help in bringing a pacified energy in the vata dosha so that the person who is going through this therapy may get peace of mind and can forget all kinds of tensions and worries which might be on their mind. The basic oil which is used during all of these therapies is sesame oil as it has a soothing effect on the body and thus helps in achieving the desired goal.

The following are some of the benefits which you will get when you opt for any of the massage therapies which have been mentioned above:

- Brings and maintains balance in all of your three doshas.

- Brings and promotes flexibility and suppleness in your body.

- Increases the level of strength and energy in your body.

- Your quality of sleep will be greatly improved.

- The softness of your skin will be greatly enhanced.

- Signs of aging will also be visibly reduced with the help of these ayurvedic therapies.

Not only this but when you opt for all or some of these kinds of therapies which belong to the ayurvedic category, then all of your stress, anxiety, and tension will disappear at once and you will be able to enjoy life to its fullest.

Chapter 4: Day By Day Easy Program to Follow

This chapter is about a day by day program which you should follow in order to lose your excess weight by using the ayurvedic way. This is a 10-day diet plan which you should follow in order to get amazing results.

How to Prepare Yourself
As you're about to start a 10-day diet plan, you should look towards preparing yourself before you actually start acting upon the 10-day diet plan. It is recommended to get yourself prepared a few days beforehand, but it is not mandatory at all. If you start preparing earlier, it will become easier for

you to act upon the diet plan for the complete ten days.

Get your mind prepared about this 10-day diet program. I must say here that this diet is comprised of vegetarian food, so when you act upon the diet plan, start to leave out the meats which you regularly consume in your current diet about two to three days before. If you are addicted to an intake of coffee, tea, sugar, or milk products, you should also start reducing the quantity of all these things from your diet about two to three days before starting the ayurvedic diet.

Food comprised of fats and junk food should also be eliminated during and sometime after the 10-day program. Keep this thing in mind when you act upon the 10-day diet plan: you are not allowed to eat any kind of food which I have mentioned above. The most important thing to consider here is if you use tobacco products or are a chain or regular smoker, then you should get rid of this habit as well in order to get the desired results of the 10-day ayurvedic diet plan.

You should not smoke or take tobacco period as it is very harmful and injurious to your health without any doubt. Another thing which is worth to consider here is that you should also stop microwaving the food you eat. Alcoholic beverages should also be eliminated during the 10-day diet plan.

Get Prepared Mentally as Well
When you are opting to act upon the ayurvedic 10-day program for weight loss, then at the initial stage, you should prepare yourself mentally as well. Before you get started with it, you should have a consultation with your physician and make sure that you don't have any ailments and you are absolutely fit to start the diet plan accordingly.

It might seem quite hard for you to stick with the same diet for a continuous ten days, but if you want to be healthy and want to lose fat, then you should listen to your body and make it your determination to do it after all.

One important aspect of this diet is that you can opt to pause or stop whenever you like. If it seems to be quite hard for you and you want to stop, you can opt to get back to your regular daily diet, but you should switch to it slowly and not suddenly.

If you face too many problems following this diet plan when you are doing it for the first time, then you can take three or four days to transition back to your normal diet. The next time you do it, you should increase the number of days going through this diet.

Diet plan

Special Herb Tea
This special tea is to be consumed about one to four cups per day.

Ingredients and Method
If you are looking to make two mugs of it then use the following quantities of ingredients. You can increase or decrease the quantity likewise.

In order to make 2 mugs of this tea, add about one fourth teaspoon of ginger powder in water. Use of dry powder is better as it is better than the fresh ginger to make your stomach work properly. Switch on the stove and boil the mixture for about four to five minutes.

It's ready now. You can make it tastier by adding a few drops of fresh lime juice to it.

Precautionary Measures
Do not over do anything with your body and listen carefully to what it wants. If you are feeling sleepy or tired, then you can add more food to your plan

so that the energy your body is looking for is fulfilled easily and without any problems.

10-Day Diet Plan
You must keep this thing in mind: While following this plan, you can eat three to four meals per day, but you should not eat more than you require in any case. For example, if you are having breakfast then most likely you should get a single serving followed by two servings for lunch and one serving for your dinner.

If you feel hungrier then you can take an additional serving between lunch and dinner. Do not let yourself go hungry for a long period of time and whenever you feel hungry, take a serving of a meal with respect to each day of your diet plan.

Each and every start of your 10-day diet should start with a glass of hot water with lemon juice in it every single morning. Do not eat or drink anything else for 10 to 15 minutes afterwards. After that, follow the diet plan.

Day 1 and 2
You should eat a bowl full of boiled vegetables along with kitchari. You can add a bit of spices, like cumin, turmeric powder, or coriander.

Recipe of Kitchari

Ingredients:
- 1 cup of split mung beans

- 1 cup basmati rice (white)

- Half tablespoon ginger, chopped

- Half a teaspoon of turmeric, cumin, and coriander powder

- A pinch of black pepper

- 6 cups of water

- Salt as required

- 2 tablespoons of ghee (clarified butter)

Directions:
- Wash and soak the beans and rice in water for about half an hour.

- Heat the water in a large pot, add the soaked beans followed by the addition of rice and all the spices. Boil everything for about 10–12 minutes.

- Now simmer the ingredients and let the mixture cook until the rice and beans become soft.

- When done, add ghee and salt just a few minutes before serving.

- If you want to turn it into a soup, then you can add about 4–5 additional cups of water and let it become frothy.

- If you just want to make mung beans then follow the same procedure as mentioned above but skip the addition of rice only.

Keep this thing in mind that the vegetables you are using may include carrots, spinach, broccoli, chard, etc.

How To Make Ghee

The traditional way to make ghee is on the stove top, but making ghee in the oven is much easier.

<u>What you need</u>:

- Approx. 1 pound of organic (450 - 500 grams) unsalted butter

- oven-safe pan

- glass container (jar)

Place the butter in the oven-safe pan. Put the pan in the oven for about 1 ½ hours at 175 degrees Fahrenheit (80 degrees Celsius).

Get a fork and skim the top, getting rid of all blemishes. Once the ghee is clean on top, pour it carefully into your glass container (jar) and leave the milky thing on the bottom out. Let it cool down and your ghee is ready!

Day 3 and 4
Eat a serving of plain kitchari without vegetables for each meal.

Day 5 and 6
For your meals, you must eat just mung bean soup without any addition of rice. But if you feel a bit hungry afterwards, you can add about a quarter cup of rice in it.

Day 7 and 8
Eat just plain kitchari without any vegetables for each meal.

Day 9 and 10
On the last two days of your diet plan, you are required to eat a bowl full of boiled vegetables along with your kitchari. Some spices can also be added to it.

When you drink water during these ten days, make sure you are drinking hot water or room temperature water. Do not drink cold water.

Triphala
It is good to take triphala, especially if you are suffering from constipation. Take 2 to 4 tablets or capsules of it at bedtime and see if your stomach is working properly in the morning.

While you are going through this 10-day diet plan, you can take triphala, which is an ayurvedic herb which consists of the formulation of the following three herbs:

- Amalaki
- Bibhitaki
- Haaritaki

Taking triphala before bed at night helps enhance the process of digestion in case it has been slowed down. This will help in the movement of your bowels one to two times more than usual in the morning.

It helps cleanse the body from the inside naturally and it's also meant for maintaining regularity. It also serves as a natural antioxidant for the body.

Initially you can take about 2 capsules of it at night but then you should increase the quantity to about 4 tablets or capsules depending how your bowel movement is in the morning. These capsules or tablets can easily be taken from any of the local herb shops near you. Then you should continue to take triphala 3 to 6 months after your 10-day detox. You can also start taking triphala a few days prior to the 10-day program.

What to Do After the 10 Days?

Once you are done with the 10-day diet plan as mentioned above, you will continue with a vegetable diet for about two to four weeks. After that, slowly incorporate chicken and fish in your meal if you like. It is highly recommended to have vegetarian food in Ayurveda, but it is not mandatory at all. To get an even better health condition, visit and consult your ayurvedic doctor or physician or a good ayurvedic health advisor on a regular basis.

Opt for Easy Exercises

When you are doing a 10-day diet plan, you must do some light and easy exercises as well like yoga, swimming, walking, etc. This will help you get your results more effectively and efficiently. You can opt for the yoga sun solution everyday just after waking up along with pranayama and meditation as well.

Chapter 5: How To Lose Weight With Ayurveda And Maintain It

You may fall in the category of those people who are very conscious about their weight and do not want to be overweight at all. At the initial stages of your life till you become 10 years old, you do not bother about your weight and anything like that, but once you become aware of how much having appropriate weight is important for you, you become conscious about it. It is not necessary that everyone remain conscious about their weight. But it can happen that when anyone starts gaining extra weight, they're more vulnerable to out of control emotions and just want to get their weight back to where it used to be.

If you have fears of gaining weight, then do not worry at all. Ayurveda has got all the solutions to the problems you are facing. You can easily cope with the weight you have gained by relying upon ayurvedic medicines because you would not have to suffer through any sort of strict activities to lose the extra weight you have gained. You can choose the way want to lose your weight. Follow the right diet and lifestyle according to your body type and you will prevent gaining weight and illness.

Why Do You Gain Weight?

According to Ayurveda, you are not advised to eat too much. You should opt for a light breakfast while lunch can be a main meal and heavy and dinner must be lighter. You should eat food to get energy and not make yourself tired due to overeating. You are recommended to avoid all cold food such as salad, sushi, raw meat, processed food, microwaved food, too much sugar, and oily and fatty foods.

There can be so many reasons behind the act which leads to having an increased body weight. Some heavy foods like dairy products and oily foods are one of the main sources that cause weight gain. You can say that the more heavy foods you sneak in your diet, the more chances you'll gain weight.

All of these heavy foods are very difficult for the body to digest and if you eat all these food items in excess then they not only work for increasing the level of heavy nutrients inside your body, but also cause the level of undigested food in the body called "ama" to increase, which is not at all good for your bodily health.

The building up of ama takes place in the digestive tract and when it causes hampering in the process of digestion, the result is the formation of variable agni which may be followed by the formation of our digestive fire which is called "dull agni." The formation of dull agni in return fires the process of metabolism which is taking place inside the body tissues. This also causes the formation of agni during the tissue metabolism as a result of which the formation of fat tissue does not happen properly and the formation of immature fat tissues takes place in more than the number which is actually required.

At the same time, when the food we eat is not getting digested properly, it will lead to the production of excess ama and eventually a vicious circle gets formed which is very difficult to be broken in case you are not aware of the way by which the stronger digestive fire can be built. But with the help of Ayurveda, you can easily cope with all the problems you have related to weight and improper digestion of food.

Now as we are talking about the ayurvedic way of losing excess weight, you have two options for it:

• Gradual weight loss

• Fast weight loss. Normally not recommended, but when detoxing the result will be fast weight loss for many. It is not recommended for people with a strong pitta dosha.

Gradual Weight Loss Option
If you feel that you have gained much weight or if you feel that the pants you wear has begun tightening, then it is the right time to make a decision about how to get rid of the excess weight you have gained. The first step which you should take is to simply avoid all oily and heavy foods, which I have mentioned earlier like dairy products and opt for all the kinds of food which are comparatively lighter. Avoid cold food and cold water.

As it is a famous principle that "like increases like," similarly when you opt for taking lighter food, you will definitely feel lighter and vice versa. The understanding of this principle is not like rocket science. It is as simple as it seems to be. All you need to have is lighter food, which will help in bringing good effects to your agni. If you are wondering what light foods are, then keep in mind that they are low-fat foods which are included in the category of light food which you should take when you are aiming to lose your weight gradually with the help of ayurvedic techniques.

The following is the list of light foods which are not only easy to be digested but also proves to be good for your agni and thus, eventually, these foods will help you in losing the excess weight you have gained so far.

Spices and Herbs
Both of these food items are not only light to eat when you are trying to lose excess weight, but they also help in bringing improvements in the digestion process. Herbs like ginger and spices like cumin, coriander, and fennel will really help you a lot in bringing improvements to your digestive system and thus help you lose the excess weight you have.

Red Lentils
They are super light and can be an important part of your diet.

Vegetables
All vegetables are light especially those which are green in color and can contribute greatly in the process of losing excess fat you have in your body.

Fruits
All fruits are light, especially apples which are stewed.

Basmati Rice
Out of all the grains, basmati rice is the lightest and most balancing one.

Point to Ponder
Now if you want to lose a small amount of weight in a gradual way, then you have to start eating foods which are comprised of vegetables and those which are heavier should be avoided completely. You can opt to have some light soups to have at dinner and in any case, the heavier meals should be avoided.

If you are looking for a way to kick start your agni to eliminate the ama which has been formed inside your body, then you can opt to have some ginger tea in the morning along with your breakfast or any other herbal tea which will definitely help you out in getting what you really want. Do not forget: drinking ginger tea is one of the most important steps of the process of starting an ayurvedic solution for losing excess weight.

Make Shifts
When you are going through the steps which have been mentioned above, you should keep this thing in mind: you can opt to work with it in simple shifts without any problems or fuss. There is no need of opting for prolonged exercises, which would leave you tired and bored of it.

Do Not Panic
Whenever you feel that you are gaining weight, then the first thing you should do is NOT panic. If you panic and worry too much, you will not be able to get your desired results. All you need to do is leave all kinds of heavy foods alone and just eat lighter foods.

Another huge benefit which you will get after going through the gradual process of losing weight through Ayurveda is that you get the desired balance of weight which you want. Once you lose the excess weight, you do not need to avoid all those heavy foods entirely. However, you should avoid those foods in great amounts, otherwise you will not be the desired weight you actually want.

Fast Weight Loss Option

If you are looking to lose your weight in a quick manner and without any problem using the ayurvedic way of treatment, then you can opt for another option which will help you achieve your desired result. This option is about losing weight in a fast manner. As far as the nature of this method is concerned, this method is almost the same as the gradual one with some slight differences. This method involves the consumption of food which is very light and should be eaten for about two weeks and then you can opt to use the gradual method for losing weight.

When I say that you are required to eat very light food during this process, I actually mean foods like moong daal, light vegetables with mixed herbs, and some light oils while you avoid all kinds of meat—whether they be white or red. Also, you are required to avoid all cold food and drinks.

These are the types of light foods which you can use during the process of losing the excess weight through the fast ayurvedic process.

- Split moong daal with light vegetable stock

- Light soup made of vegetables

- Split moong daal made with a greater quantity of water

- Stir-fried vegetables

- Pancakes made of moong daal

How Can You Help Your Agni?
You can help your agni, the digestive fire, by getting rid of excess ama which has been produced inside your body. You can get rid of this ama by drinking a cup of ginger tea two times a day, especially in the morning before eating breakfast. This will help you get rid of all the undigested food which is inside your body due to poor digestion. Or you can drink ginger tea half an hour before every meal or after every meal for digestion.

The fast option of losing weight using light food helps you lose weight by firing your agni and by reducing the amount of ama, which has been produced inside your body, but these processes can only be kept going for a shorter period of time. While you are going through the process of losing weight in a fast manner, you are required to not even look at heavy foods and avoid them for every meal, every day.

If you are looking to lose a larger amount of weight which you have gained in a very short interval of time, then you are required to mix up both of the approaches—gradual and fast. If you use both approaches, then in the first two weeks you would start off with the fast approach and then switch to the gradual approach for an additional two weeks.

The combined effect of both options has proven to be very cumulative as far as the cleansing effect of both is concerned. This is a kind of therapy which is associated with the ayurvedic way of treating the problem of weight loss without any difficulty. Keep this in mind that when you are opting for the ayurvedic ways of losing weight, you are required to get rid of ama as much as you can so that the harmful effects of ama cannot provide harm to you in any way. Getting rid of excess ama is a major step in losing the excess weight which you have gained.

Consider Your Lifestyle
You can also feel heavy when you have a sedentary lifestyle. In addition to the previous ayurvedic approaches to losing weight, you are also required to do exercise on a daily basis so that you don't feel any sort of problems in losing the excess weight which you have gained. This is especially important when you are thinking of doing the fast

option; you are definitely required to do exercise with it because without it, the fast option would not have the results you desire.

Opt for Exercise

Doing exercise on a daily basis does not mean that you are required to do a heavy drill every single day. Just a light drill of about 10–15 minutes daily is enough for you to live a healthy life. The exercises which can be done on a daily basis to lose weight include: yoga, brisk walking, tai chi, swimming, and much more. All of these exercises would definitely help you out in lightening your heaviness and in firing up your agni and, ultimately, bring down the level of ama from your body so that you can live healthy and without any problems of gaining excess weight again and again.

If you are working with the gradual option of losing weight, then you can do something more than this as well. In gradual weight loss you are required to keep yourself motivated by sticking to an exercise as a habit. Yes, you should take up an exercise as a habit and this habit should be continued even after losing your excess weight as it will help you out in maintaining your body at a normal level even when you have reached your desired weight.

Sleeping Should Be Limited

If you sleep just after eating your meal, then it will have a great negative impact on not only your stomach, but on your overall bodily health. So you should avoid getting up late and you should try to get up early in the morning. This will ensure that the harmful effects of sleeping late at night and getting up late in the morning be minimized to a great extent.

Fulfilling 8 hours of sleep is mandatory. If you were not able to sleep earlier at night then you can cover the missed sleeping hours in the afternoon the next day. This will help you create a healthy lifestyle and thus help you get rid of any health problems which you might be suffering from.

So the ayurvedic secret of losing weight is just comprised of two simple methods and it is totally up to you which method you want to use to lose the excess weight you have. These approaches will help look after your agni, which is not possible in any other kind of dietary or weight loss plan which you use in order to lose the excess amount of fat which has accumulated inside your body. Other diets only focus on minimizing the amount of ama inside your body.

Do not think that the ayurvedic approach is just a weight loss approach. The fact is, it is a complete approach which can be referred to as a preventive health approach as it really helps you look after the agni which is in your gut and also the agni which resides in your liver and tissues and are working on preventing the production of ama inside your body. Not only this, but the ayurvedic approach of losing weight also helps you bring balance to the doshas you have, thus helping you prevent the onset of some diseases which are chronic in nature and should be avoided in all cases.

Conclusion

Thank you again for buying this book!

Using the ayurvedic way of treating various health-related problems will help you get rid of these problems without putting any extra effort. Use of ayurvedic medicines is actually based on a theory which is about the universe and its elements. This theory gives great emphasis on everything which is related to the natural remedies of anything. In addition to improving the health of the mind and soul, ayurvedic medicines also help in losing weight.

You can get a lot of benefits out of Ayurveda if you have a complete set of knowledge about everything related to Ayurveda and ayurvedic medicines. The entire process by which your body works and its constitution comes out by the combination of physical and psychological attributes which come under the heading of prakriti. The basic goal of opting for the ayurvedic way of healing any ailment is to bring balance in your body so that you can be able to get rid of all the problems which are related to your health. The integration of all of the functions that are being carried out inside your body can also be enhanced by using ayurvedic powers.

Ayurveda is comprised of five basic elements and when they combine together, they form a well-balanced combination which is essential for properly implementing the process of Ayurveda to your body. It can be said that the five systems of Ayurveda is a complete system by which the importance of ayurvedic medicines can be taken into consideration very easily and all of these elements in combination with one another help in gaining many benefits which is unimaginable.

As the basic origin of ayurvedic medicines is from India, the various terminologies which have been used throughout this book related to Ayurveda have a Sanskrit origin and most of the words are spoken in the Hindi language. One of the important goals of opting for ayurvedic medicines is that this method, in addition to various other benefits, also helps in optimizing your health. And not just your physical health, but your mental health will also be improved with the help of using ayurvedic medicines.

All the related information regarding Ayurveda and ayurvedic medicines has been added in this book and I hope it will really help you get rid of any health-related problem you have. Whether you want to lose weight or if you are looking for some remedy to restore your digestive system, all you need is to follow the steps and information which has been given in this book. All of the information will really help you out in getting what you want.

You have also learnt the basic information about Ayurveda and its related medicines and I hope that if you had been looking for a way to lose your excess weight or to detoxify your body that you would consider using the golden principles of Ayurveda, which have been mentioned in this book.

Finally, if you enjoyed this book, then I'd like to ask you for a favor. Would you be kind enough to leave a review for this book on Amazon? It'd be greatly appreciated!

Thank you and good luck!

Michael Dinuri

www.dinuri.com

About the Author

Michael Dinuri is a Swedish Ayurveda, yoga, and Vaastu practitioner and author. Dinuri has always believed that life has unlimited possibilities to offer and he is passionate about helping other people change their lives and share his knowledge. As a result, he is now able to professionally work with personal development and wellness.

Dinuri's grandparents originated from northwest India, a country where yoga and alternative medicine has been used since ancient times and is still commonly used in everyday life. At an early age, encouraged and inspired by his paternal grandmother, he became intrigued by the infinite ancient knowledge and wisdom of human life and nature.

A lot of Dinuri's knowledge has been obtained through the studies of ancient scriptures and by being a disciple of well-known teachers and masters of India and other parts of the world. Dinuri also has a vast interest in mysticism and has a passion for fulfilling everyone's potential as a human being.

"The key to the road of happiness is to learn how to understand our inner being, and in doing so, be able to enjoy our every moment to the fullest."

— Michael Dinuri

Other books by Michael Dinuri:

Meditation

The Ultimate and Easy Guide to Learn How to Be Peaceful and Relieve Stress, Anxiety And Depression

— By Michael Dinuri

Meditation is a lifestyle skill that brings not only peacefulness to the person practicing the skill, but also provides lifelong health benefits that add longevity and quality of life. It is a simple skill that can be practiced by anyone of any age, race, religion, political view point, or regional location with no special requirements or equipment needed.

This book will cover not only the benefits from a regular meditation schedule, but will also provide tips for short, easy to use, mini meditations for those on-the-go days when you just need a break from the harsh realities of everyday living

Vastu Secrets in Modern Times for A Successful Life
Improve Your Health, Wealth And Relationships With Indian Feng Shui

— By Michael Dinuri

Vastu Shastra is the art of arranging your home or work place to work in harmony with the flow of energy that surrounds us on a daily basis and to mimic nature in such a way as to honor it. Much like the Chinese art of Feng Shui, Vastu Shastra is becoming an integral part of everyday life for millions of people around the world. When we invest time in our homes and our personal well-being, there are bound to be positive effects with long reaching benefits that bring happiness and peace to our lives.

Vastu Shastra may have originated many years ago in India, however, the lessons it teaches are timeless and especially important in the current high-stress society that we live in today. Vastu wisdom teaches us to reunite with the forces of the universe to achieve personal wealth, health, and happiness on a variety of levels that can only happen once we have acknowledged and honored the endless energies that flow through our lives at any given time.

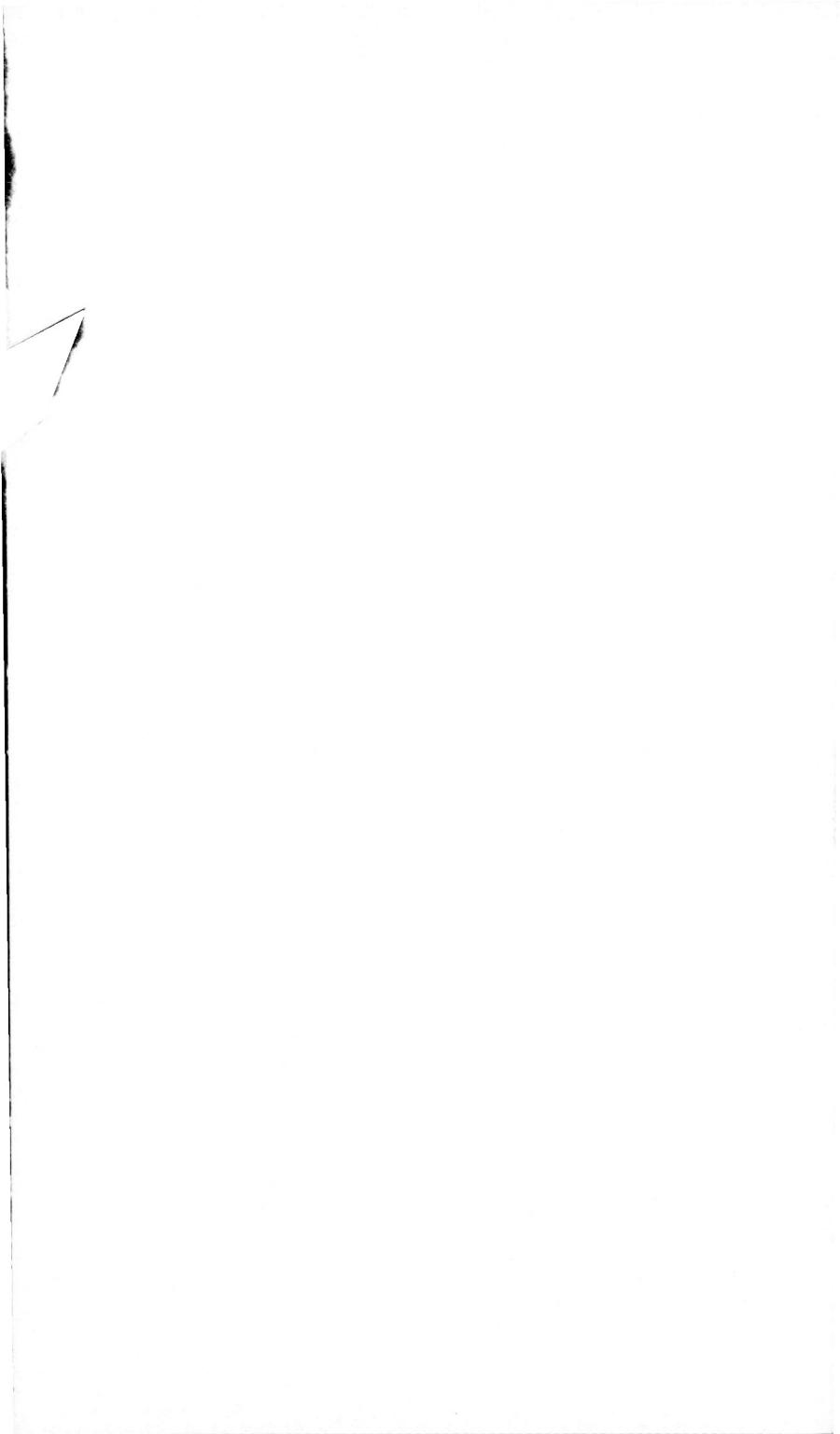

Printed in Great Britain
by Amazon